The Friendly Handbook of Shoulder Surgery Coping Tips

and Tricks

Patients Talk about Managing after Shoulder Replacement

and Rotator Cuff Repair

by

Bruce H. Wolk

First Printing, 2018

ISBN-13: 978-1985884762

Bruce H. Wolk
Made Here Books, LLC
Denver, Colorado 80220

Contents

Introduction

Hello from a Real Patient,

In 2017, there were about 53,000 total shoulder replacement surgeries in the U.S. (up from only 18,000 in 2000), about 272,000 rotator cuff repairs and 258,000 shoulder arthroscopies (more than a 70 percent increase from 2007). The number of patients having all types of shoulder surgeries is growing each year.

In interviewing shoulder replacement and rotator cuff patients about how they came to have shoulder problems, the top reasons mentioned were: *job-related injuries, accidents, falls* and *arthritis*. I am "proud" to say that I fell into all of these categories.

My shoulder got slammed around a great deal when I was a New York City paramedic, including one eventful evening when the ambulance overturned!

A year later, just walking my dog, I took a hard fall on an icy sidewalk, and over time I developed painful arthritis in the shoulder.

About 12 years prior to the total shoulder replacement, I had an arthroscopy; I was "scoped" to remove bone chips and to help me with the arthritis. At that time, the orthopedic surgeon said that I would eventually need a total shoulder replacement. He was right, though I didn't want him to be right.

Last year, the pain became too much to bear. My workouts were excruciating and I could no longer sleep. At the behest of friends, I tried many non-invasive approaches from acupuncture, physical therapy and chi gung to glucosamine, vitamins and dietary changes. My shoulder was finished and I accepted that the only remaining choice was surgery.

Prior to the shoulder replacement surgery, I heard that any kind of shoulder procedure may initially alter how we sleep, how we manage personal hygiene, how we travel, dress, exercise and even prepare our meals. I heard that recovery could take months and, in some cases, it could take up to a year or more to restore strength and function. I was to learn that "hearing" and "experiencing" were two very different things.

Sitting at My Desk (Writing One-Handed)

As I am writing this introduction I am still wearing my sling. It has been six and a half weeks since I had a total shoulder replacement surgery. This week I am scheduled to begin life without the sling. I am in physical therapy twice a week. I also exercise at home.

Before I scare anyone away from having surgery, I need to say something that I think is important. My pain level after nearly seven weeks post-op is just a fraction of what it was prior to surgery.

My range of motion is improving with each week and my physical therapist is pleased with my progress. I do not regret that I had it done. Most shoulder surgery patients I interviewed felt the same way.

Now What?

Whether you are facing a total shoulder replacement, a partial shoulder replacement, reverse shoulder replacement, the many types of rotator cuff repair or any number of combinations of those procedures (for example, a total shoulder replacement also includes surgical procedures to the rotator cuff), the biggest challenges will come after the surgery and during the first weeks and months of recovery.

During those first days, weeks and months you are basically down to using one arm. It is an awkward time and often a frustrating one.

No one talks about just how frustrating coping with one arm can be and that is why I decided to start this book while I'm going through the daily chores of living it myself.

Orthopedic surgeons do their jobs well, but after your procedure, they are on to the next patient. It's the nature of things. There is little time for chit-chat. I am not faulting them; they are in business. However, understand that most orthopedic surgeons, their assistants, orthopedic nurses, technicians and physical therapists *have never had* shoulder surgery themselves. They have little hands-on knowledge for coping with everyday nuisances and painful realities.

The attitude among most in the medical community is that patients will figure things out on their own. Well, that's a lot of figuring out. There are always new challenges and minor inconveniences and this book aims to help you with them.

11

Those who can best answer your coping questions are other patients, those of us who have had to figure things out for ourselves.

One afternoon, not long after surgery, I was walking around the block to get some fresh air. I was in my sling. A stranger was walking in the other direction.

"Rotator cuff?" she asked.

I told her it was a total shoulder replacement. She shared that she had had rotator cuff repair about a year before. We started talking and she began to share tips about how she learned to put on shoes with one hand! Shoulder surgery patients are like that. I have found them to be quite kind and considerate.

The Friendly Handbook of Shoulder Surgery Coping Tips and Tricks reflects the need that shoulder surgery patients have to share. I know there are other references available, but they are either "scientific" or limited to a single, personal experience.

In writing this book, I decided to take a different approach — this book is written in forum-like fashion. I quote patients as though they are in a large lecture hall comparing notes and talking to one another.

Scope of This Book

The Friendly Handbook of Shoulder Surgery Coping Tips and Tricks is based on first-person interviews, email and snail mail correspondence, stories and the observations of fellow patients. *You will be reading their actual words.* However, the names have been "scrambled" and altered. There is one exception to the rule: me! My initials, "BHW," appear after my quotes.

The Friendly Handbook of Shoulder Surgery Coping Tips and Tricks gives practical advice as to how patients coped with shoulder surgeries in the first few days, weeks and months. The advice ranges from meal preparation and dog walking to how women dealt with their underwear.

Some of the quotes are intimate, some are funny. As you read through the comments, my hope is that you will come away with some good ideas. I don't expect that all of the experiences will apply to everyone, but I have already applied some of them myself.

This book *does not discuss* pain-killing or anti-inflammatory medications, medical symptoms or pre- or post-surgical problems.

You are strongly urged to contact your medical provider about any medical concerns.

A gentle warning about social media support groups: Most of those in the groups really are supportive, but occasionally you will run into a "know-it-all doctor" who has never seen the inside of a medical school. *Please steer clear* of anyone who dispenses medical, surgical or pharmaceutical advice on a social media website. Please don't let a stranger play amateur orthopedic surgeon with you.

Don't let a social media friend diagnose you or read your MRI. If you are in pain or you are having a reaction of any kind, immediately call your healthcare provider.

Don't Judge

Don't judge your progress against anyone else's progress, and don't grow impatient with yourself. The shoulder is a complex joint. Healing takes time. We all have good days and lousy days. It is not a straight line from surgery to complete healing — it is more like a wave. Some days you will feel as though you're at the top of the mountain; other days you will be in the valley.

If it hurts to do something, *don't do it* or back off and do it again slowly. Pain is personal, as is every surgical procedure. If you are concerned about something, call your surgeon's office and get help.

1. Basic Principles

Thinking Ahead

Most of us were born with the blessing of having two arms and two legs. When we have one of those limbs temporarily knocked out of commission as the result of a surgical procedure or injury, we come to realize how much we rely on that "missing limb" in daily use.

When a procedure is done to our shoulder, either the dominant or non-dominant arm, it immediately throws us off. In the case of a shoulder, it is not just the shoulder, it is also our arm and hand.

It is common sense that having a shoulder procedure immediately affects our strength in that arm. We lose that strength quickly, especially when we are immobilized in a sling.

After shoulder surgery, we must learn to slowly strengthen that arm and expand its range of motion. In addition, we must guard against injuring it during the healing process. Treat yourself with kindness. In thinking ahead, we need to reason with our condition in terms of "Healing and Guarding." In fact, our prime mission is to heal.

Don't Push It!

I have interviewed people who sheepishly told me they "pushed things too hard," intentionally ignoring doctors' orders. Somehow, the words "wimp," "whiner" or "weakling" always like to surface! No one, it seems, female or male, wants to be seen as anything less than strong, stoic and super-human. The "tough guy" mindset always winds up causing patients trouble. For example, if a surgeon recommends that a patient should stay in a sling for the better part of six weeks, and the patient decides after one week that they "don't need that stupid sling," there's no one to blame but themselves if something goes wrong.

A shoulder surgery patient must always keep in mind whether what they are doing will help the shoulder to heal or if it will potentially make the shoulder more painful or lengthen the healing. Let it heal, guard against hurting it. If you can't decide whether you should push something or not, ask yourself, "What's the kindest thing?" Follow that instinct.

Thinking Ahead

If you're in a sling, thinking ahead involves protecting the healing arm in all kinds of situations. Most of us go through life on automatic. We do things, and we don't spend a lot of time thinking about them.

In talking to physical therapists, I have learned that *the most common way patients re-injure their shoulders is from falls.*

No one can plan for everything in life, but by thinking ahead for those first weeks, you can drastically cut down the chances of falling.

It will be necessary to think ahead when you're at a crowded party or out with a group of people, when first sitting down or arising from an unstable chair, when walking up and down a flight of stairs and when moving along a walkway in an airport or riding an escalator.

If you're in a sling, think ahead when getting into a vehicle, crossing a busy intersection, or going into a jammed store or restaurant. Think ahead when reaching for something on a shelf or walking in the dark around a theater or sports stadium.

I am not saying you should be afraid of anything and everything, just honor your health. In those first days and weeks after shoulder surgery, your balance and way of moving can be off.

Many intentionally wear their sling even after their surgeons say it is OK to go without it in crowded situations to serve as a kind of warning to others.

The people who have gone through what you are about to go through all agree that "thinking ahead" will become second nature. It is just a matter of being aware.

I might add a word or two about alcohol. Be especially cautious about drinking or being around others who are drinking to excess when you are wearing a sling.

True story from someone I corresponded with on Facebook: He was at a Christmas party, wearing a sling about a month after rotator cuff surgery. A tipsy relative thought it would be cute to playfully punch him in his arm. He was in so much pain after the punch, he had to sit down. The relative offered a slurred apology after others screamed at her. For about an hour, he was terrified he would have to return to surgery. Fortunately, she missed the incision.

Caution is smarter than re-injury. Be very aware of everything. You are on no timetable except your own. Be kind, think ahead, and don't rush it.

Keep It in Balance

"I have an inner ear disease (Meniere's) that used to badly affect my balance. The dizziness usually doesn't bother me anymore, but after surgery I was pretty wobbly from the medication. I reminded myself to be careful. I was prepared for anything that came along. After a day or two it passed." – Bob B.

What is not so clear before shoulder surgery is that when the arm and hand are in a sling, even the best of us may have our balance affected. It may be just a little inconvenience for some and a big deal for others.

"Keeping it in balance" is something to consider when we are thinking ahead.

For example, if we are recovering from surgery and there are snowy or icy conditions, we must be careful when we go out. Black ice (invisible ice on a road or sidewalk) can be a huge problem. The same hazard may also be present when we walk on wet grass or leaves. But it is not just snow, ice, grass or even artificial turf. There are many more potential dangers to our balance when we're in that sling.

Shower stalls and bathtubs can be dangerous places, especially if we're in any kind of sling. So are garden centers, wet floors in supermarkets or department stores and the slick floors of airports, train stations, bus terminals and subways.

Uneven surfaces can be a problem, such as going from carpet to a waxed wood floor or slick tile. Cords and wires on the floor are potential tripping hazards, as are pet toys (and pets!), kids' toys, sporting equipment, plant stands, cushions and furniture.

"I got up from the recliner in the middle of the night to use the bathroom. This was in my own living room. I was wearing the sling so I was off-balance. My foot 'hooked' on a cushion and I came within an inch of a huge fall right on the surgical shoulder." – Jan S.

Before surgery, think ahead as to what you can do in your home to lessen balance problems after surgery. Just as you might child-proof or puppy-proof your home, think in terms of shoulder-proofing.

"I went into a panic the other day. I was in my sling. I sat down in my new recliner for the first time and leaned over too far and I felt it tipping. Scared me to death. This is not a good feeling when you have had a knee operation and two replaced shoulder joints!" – Barb L.

Give serious thought to potential balance problems, even if you don't ordinarily have them. Don't create problems for yourself.

For example, do you love to ride your bicycle? Using a reclining bike in the gym or in your home to maintain cardio makes a lot of sense; riding around the neighborhood while in a sling makes no sense at all. Stay off the treadmill too. It is very easy to get off balance. Do you love yoga? Great! Unless you're a master, try more stable poses until you're far along in healing. The same is true with tai chi or dance. Don't be ruled by ego. There is plenty of time to regain form.

"You know, I finally went back to playing tennis at about eight months after my shoulder replacement operation but actually it took at least another four months, so about a year, for me to regain my full strength and have my full range of motion kick in.... You can't rush it." – Janie J.

2. The Three-Legged Stool

An image you might find helpful is that of a low, three-legged stool, an old-fashioned three-legged wooden milking stool. What makes the three-legged stool interesting for our shoulder surgery conversation is that it is *low*, *strong* and *stable*. Think of your body in a sling in the same way. After surgery, the lower you keep your center of gravity when you are dressing, eating, showering, etc., the better.

For example, in the first days and weeks, when you have just finished showering and you are attempting to put on underwear or socks, the more you can do those activities in a seated position, the more stable you are.

I have spoken to some patients who in the very beginning usually sat when putting on slacks or trousers.

They briefly stood to hike up the slacks and then they fastened them while laying down on a bed or couch. The more stable you can be, the better.

While in a sling, sitting on a chair is more stable than on a high stool. While in a sling, eating while standing is less stable than eating while sitting.

Keep it low, keep it safe.

Practice

Leading up to surgery, it is a good idea to practice everyday tasks with the one good arm and hand to get used to being "one-handed." It won't exactly duplicate how you will feel after surgery, but it's a start.

BUT! There is a hidden danger in practicing with one arm that I personally learned about the hard way. Be aware that you can hurt or strain the good arm by rushing, lifting too much and basic overuse.

The dumb mistake I made was in overpacking my gym bag and yanking it straight off the floor and above my head to stick it in a locker. That one dumb move caused a muscle strain that lasted for weeks.

In interviewing other shoulder replacement and rotator cuff patients, they also reported similar "strains and pains" problems from asking the good arm and shoulder to do everything. Immediately going from two arms to one is not without its risks. You are asking the non-surgical arm and shoulder to do a lot — sometimes, too much. Be gentle with your "good arm" as you recover. Slow but sure, the two arms will again be balanced in the workload, but it will take time.

Practicing everyday tasks with one arm is positive, but straining that arm doing everything accomplishes nothing.

One additional point is important to mention, and that is "reflexive action."

Before surgery, you went through life with those two arms and those cat-like reflexes (or so you thought). You reacted to near drops, near misses, near falls and other "oops" moments, and you amazed your friends as you caught dishes or a tipped glass.

You will not lose the memory of those reflexive actions when you are in a sling. If you move too quickly and drop something or an object slips, your reflexes will kick in and you may experience some discomfort in the jerking motion. While we can't anticipate accidents, your fellow patients would again tell you to move deliberately to guard against discomfort or injury.

Get Help

"I have the best neighbors in the world. I had my shoulder surgery done at the start of winter and my neighbor Scott shoveled my walk all the way through. He said, 'That's what neighbors are for!'" – Diana C.

Many of us are taught from small-fry to be self-reliant and independent. We grow into adults often thinking we don't need help. Whether unfortunate or not, having any kind of shoulder surgery forces us to rely on family, friends and strangers for support.

"I got into arguments with my wife because she wanted to help me do stuff and I wanted to be my usual stubborn self. I quickly realized I needed help. I had a full-thickness rotator cuff repair. I couldn't do it alone. Looking back, I think it's a good thing to ask for help. Sometimes it's OK to be weak." – Carl T.

If you live alone, you need to develop some kind of network to help you with household tasks, meal preparation, socializing and driving. Whether this network involves a home aide, a cook, nursing care or light house cleaning is difficult to say, but if you need some help those first days and weeks, you should not be afraid to ask for it if for no other reason than being immobilized in a sling could put you off-balance.

If you have had physical problems prior to shoulder surgery, that is all the more reason to get help. For example, if you have had back, hip, knee or foot surgery (as have many of the older shoulder surgery patients I interviewed), you may already have moderate difficulty moving. Being immobilized in a sling and having reduced strength in one arm or leg or your back is really expecting your body to do a great deal on its own.

There comes a time when it is important to ask for help — you needn't be a hero or "she-ro" all of the time.

"Believe it or not, my shoulder surgery brought us closer. My husband turned out to be a decent cook after all! He really came through. I can't say he'll open up a restaurant, but he enjoyed cooking. He got a kick out of serving me while I was recuperating — he even admitted it!" – Regina H.

3. Sleeping Tips and Tricks

We all know that sleeping is fundamental to wellness. In fact, many total shoulder replacement and rotator cuff patients reported that it was the lack of sleep brought on by the pain that finally drove them to have surgery. Many patients told me that it was not until after they had surgery that they had their first decent sleep in months.

However, sleeping with a newly repaired shoulder brings on problems of its own. As the shoulder begins its healing process, it may be difficult to find a comfortable sleeping position. No medical professionals seem to want to talk about this, but your fellow shoulder patients will! Many change the way they sleep in the weeks following shoulder surgery.

It is almost a guarantee that you will need to be elevated *in some way* to take pressure off of your shoulder repair or replacement. Every shoulder surgery patient I personally encountered had discomfort in trying to sleep "flat."

After surgery, the trick is to take pressure off the shoulder joint and/or its surrounding muscles. For some, it may take up to six months *or more* to sleep in a "normal" way.

In general, the sleeping tips and tricks the patients spoke about regarding comfort fell into three broad areas:

a. **Reclining Chairs** - Using either a reclining chair or a bed that reclines,

b. **Wedge** - Using a foam wedge plus pillows to elevate the body in the bed,

c. **Pillows** - Modifying the bed by loading it up with pillows of all sorts until there is adequate support and comfort.

There is no right or wrong sleeping solution, but be aware of what they all have in common: the need for *comfort and elevation.*

The following are some tips your fellow "slingers" want to share with you about how they got decent sleep. I have arranged these tips and tricks as three separate "forums."

Reclining Chairs

Far and away, reclining chairs were reported to be the most comfortable way to sleep for those who were recovering from shoulder procedures. Owned, borrowed or rented, recliners provided support and relief even for those who were not normally back sleepers. One important point all mentioned was that if you do decide to use a recliner, *use an electric one,* not a manual one.

The length of time the recliners were used could range from a few days to seven months or more.

33

Those who were loyal to recliners had the following things to say:

"By all means, if you have the money, buy an inexpensive recliner and get used to it before surgery. My reclining chair 'saved my life!' I used it to sleep for two months steady, then slowly eased off of it over the next two months. When I was recovering from my TSR it took all of the pressure off my shoulder. I got a recliner with an electrical motor which was much better than a mechanical arm and not too much more expensive. You can also rent one pretty cheaply. If you have a good friend who has a recliner, you can always try talking them into loaning it to you. I wound up giving mine to a friend who had rotator cuff surgery." – Harlan W.

"I recommend a reclining chair but it depends on sleeping arrangements in your house. If you share a bed with someone, definitely use a recliner.

When I was by myself, I used about five pillows stacked on top of each other and leaned up against the headboard. That way you have more control of arranging the support of your back and head. But when I wasn't alone, I went back to the recliner." – Carol

"I had a reverse shoulder replacement. I am now at 14 weeks recovery and still sleeping in a recliner. I cannot lay down for more than 45 minutes in a bed. I have not found the correct pillow placement yet." – Jane

"Not exactly a recliner, but I have an adjustable bed base that I can put in a sitting position, and I was in that position for about 10 weeks with a pillow under my arm." – Peter M.

"Oh yes, I was in a recliner for about a month and a half before I attempted to sleep in my bed." – Lisa G.

"I slept in my recliner for two days to keep the pressure off of my shoulder and then I was able to sleep slightly elevated on pillows in my bed." – Scott R.

"Here's how I used the recliner after surgery — I put pillows on either side of my body and head, kind of like 'bumper pillows.' I put the recliner against the wall so [I could] lean [my] non-surgical side against the pillow." – Pam

"I am now at seven weeks post rotator cuff surgery. Still sleeping on a chaise lounge. I tried our recliner but at first, didn't realize the [mechanical] lever was on my surgery side. I had to get my husband to release it, so I was completely stuck if he wasn't around." – June P.

"I'm now seven months out of surgery. I try to sleep in the bed but I still use my recliner when my shoulder muscles start aching after a tough physical therapy session or pushing myself a little harder in the gym." – Elke B.

"I should have gotten an electric recliner, even one with a remote control. I wasn't thinking so I had my daughter stuff a pillow under the manual lever so it couldn't latch.

It made it so much easier to be independent and not to have someone recline me every time I got up." – Hans B.

"I had to work my way back into my bed. An hour in the bed with my sling on, then back to the recliner or the couch. I would try to extend the time in bed a little longer and then back into bed without the sling with lots of pillows for positioning." – Oren R.

"Unfortunately, I haven't slept in a bed in over seven months, the recliner is just easier." – CF

"This shoulder surgery [it was his second], *it was about three and a half weeks in the recliner before I could sleep in my bed. I just could not stand the recliner a moment longer, but it was necessary."* – Ben R.

"I bought what is called a powered 'lift recliner' that tilts up and forward to meet you. It can flatten out to make a great bed or it can adjust in many ways to fit my spine. When I am sleeping, if I want to vary the curvature it does so perfectly." – Robert

"I am two weeks post op for total shoulder replacement surgery. I tried to sleep in my bed last night with the sling on and a pillow under it. It was a lot of work getting adjusted and it hurt. I tried to force myself to try it for a few hours. I ended up back in the chair for a total of two hours of sleep. Guess I'm not ready for the bed yet. Pretty disappointed." – Marti P.

"I tried a foam wedge 'pillow' the other night and built it up with several pillows. I slept for a few minutes and said to myself, 'Nope, it's not going to happen.' I went back to the recliner. Then last night I used the wedge and went down to one pillow and finally slept. You've got to experiment." – ABV

"In my opinion you're going to have to choose between a recliner and a wedge pillow. It's extremely painful to lay flat. You won't be sleeping on your side after the operation. Also, pillows shift in the night. I like being stable." – Alan A.

Wedges

After the recliner, many shoulder surgery patients preferred the use of a foam wedge in a bed to elevate and take pressure off of their shoulder. Foam wedges are easy to source online and they are widely available in pharmacies, sporting goods stores and medical supply stores. They are (obviously) easier to store and cheaper to buy than a recliner. Wedges provide good support. They may be used with or without pillows.

"After my cuff repair, I always slept in the bed, but I used a foam wedge and lots of pillows for a week or two post-op." – KMG

"As I was recovering, I was very comfortable leaning against a large wedge cushion on my bed with two pillows on top of it and other pillows supporting my arm." – Linda H.

"I always slept in my own bed. I was not tempted to buy a recliner, but I had a foam wedge with lots of pillows on it for a week or two post-op. I gradually worked my way back down until I could sleep flat. Some nights during healing, the pain from sleeping flat came back to my shoulder and I put the wedge back on." – JMS

"I found a wedge for side sleeping. There are several companies who make orthopedic pillow supports. They're not that expensive. Why be miserable?" – Gil J.

"I slept in a recliner the first few weeks. Then I tried sleeping in my bed with lots of pillows and I was tired and miserable. I bought a wedge pillow online and I sleep well on that. I'm about 10 weeks post-op and I still can't sleep without elevation." – BJ

Modifying a Bed or Couch with Pillows

Using a pile of pillows or one big body pillow with smaller pillows may or may not be easier — or cheaper — than a wedge.

Pillows seemed a more transitional method to achieve comfort for most patients as they went from a recliner or wedge to a flat bed. On the other hand, large pillows may be used long after your shoulder has improved as part of your décor or to help you exercise. Those who were loyal to pillow arrangements had the following things to say:

"The body pillow I ordered will help me do my floor stretches and may help me to sleep in the bed. I don't know if I'll still need the foam wedge from time to time." – Patricia

"Get a memory foam pillow. At first, I bought another kind but it turned out to be too big for my neck, so I use it in my pickup to prop up my arm." – Brian

"I found a memory foam pillow with other pillows to be very effective. I used a half-moon shape bolster." – Anonymous

"I am a side-sleeper, always have been. I spent several lousy nights in a recliner until I finally gave up. I got into bed and my wife propped pillows around me until I was comfortable. You need to see what's best for you." – Eric

"I just used the decorative pillows off of my couch. They are very flexible and I could fit them between my chin and shoulder as my head wanted to tilt to the side." – JC

"The first night after my surgery my wife got me one of those neck pillows. It was a huge help." – Alan F.

"You can go back to your bed and sleeping flat when you are comfortable but it takes time. For me, I needed a pile of comfy pillows on top of the upright, or 'bed rest' pillow. That method worked best for me. I was able to almost sleep normally after about 10 days. Pain is very personal." – Samantha

"I bought a pillow called the 'Flex 4-in-1 travel pillow.'

I think any neck pillow will help save you from throwing out your neck or back when you're propped up with a sling. " – Bill T.

"*Several companies make an adjustable backrest. They are lightweight and can be set up on the bed. You will probably need to pile pillows up against it. It's a good alternative to a bed rest pillow because it can change positions.* " – Al

"*I transitioned from the recliner to the bed after eight weeks. I used two pillows and a neck pillow and I supported my surgical shoulder with a small Japanese-type rice-hull pillow. Every so often the pillows slip [so] you're lying flat and pain returns to the shoulder.* " – BHW

"*I'm seven weeks post-op and I can now sleep in a bed. Even though I'm asleep, I'm aware of where my arm is. I keep a pillow under my surgical arm. It's not easy, but I'm done with the recliner.* " – John L.

"I tried laying on my non-surgical side in the beginning, but my surgical side felt very awkward and painful even though there was no pressure on it. The bolster on the sling was cumbersome. I went back to putting a cushy pillow under my arm to keep it in place. Then you have the period when the bolster is removed and there's another adjustment to go through. You're going to have to experiment." – Carol D.

"I'm using two body pillows, one for each side of my body, and a foam orthopedic neck pillow. The neck pillow is a half-circle and it's made of memory foam." – PC

"I just found a U-shaped body pillow that I really liked a lot. It is also described as a pregnancy pillow but it has many uses. It surrounds my body [and] elevates and supports my shoulder. There are several manufacturers who make them at a good price." – Meghan B.

"For me, the recliner wasn't too comfy. There're some good ones for sure, but not mine. So, the first night I used like 100 pillows every which way to prop me up and to stabilize. Over time I cut back on the pillows." – SS

"I hate sleeping in the recliner! I was a week post-op and my back and neck became sore and irritated. I have found my neck pillow to be very helpful." – Leon

"From day one, I used a lot of pillows to prop me up and support my arms and under my knees, and that way I could be in my own room and have my own TV and my own AC. I could close my door and slept whenever I needed to do so." – Nancy B.

Sleep Safety Tips

Awakening in the night and needing to get out of a recliner, couch or bed carries risks not encountered before surgery.

Balance and disorientation may be problems, unfamiliarity with where you are sleeping may result in accidents, tripping hazards may be present. There are steps that can be taken to avoid accidents.

Night Lights

"I strongly recommend night lights for any room you sleep in and also for the bathroom. Night lights cost what? Just about nothing. If you're in a sling and the anesthesia is wearing off, you're going to get confused or maybe trip over a wire or a pillow or something in the middle of the night." – Harold W.

"Install switches with lighting in all of the critical rooms. The 'night light wall switches' are easy to install and any electrician or handyman can install them in no time at all. I put them in my kitchen, bathroom and living room because I had my recliner set up there." – Frank

"Remember those 'Clapper Lights' we used to joke about? They still make them and they work! If you or

someone in the family has just had surgery, you can rig the unit up to any light near the recliner or bed for safety." – Sharon M.

Glasses and Cups
"Wouldn't you know it, I'm such a klutz! I usually bring a glass of water into the bedroom at night and place it on my nightstand. I think it was my second night after surgery that the glass slipped out of my hand and fell on the floor. I had pieces of glass all over the floor which was hard to clean up with the sling on. From then on, I put everything in plastic." – Craig

"It's a lot easier to have plastic cups with tops and straws. Really cuts down on spills in the middle of the night." – Kathy

Cords
"Controls to electric blankets should be off the floor, so you can make changes to the settings easier." – Gabe

"Blinds, shades and curtains have cords and they can be hazards if you don't know where you're walking."

"I never used an alarm clock because of the cords and inconvenience. I used my cell phone for my alarms." – Harold

Take a Tour

"When you decide where you want to sleep, after you set everything up the way you want, make the room as dark as possible and then walk around. Get used to it. If you trip over anything or bump into anything, take care of it right away." – Shelley G.

"If you got kids or grandkids or a sloppy husband (lol), lay down the law! Nothing on the floor like magazines, clothes, shoes, a rubber ball or a toy. Best of luck!" – Marcia S.

4. Relaxation/ Alternatives to Pain Management

Given the current concerns over painkillers, several patients offered that they used meditation and relaxation techniques rather than medication to control pain in the weeks following surgery. Pain is a personal challenge and pain management falls outside the scope of this handbook. Nevertheless, people volunteered their thoughts on the topic and they are worth sharing.

"Remember to 'keep breathing,' and when you feel all tense, make sure to take deep, long breaths and relax your jaw. Keep paying attention to your breath and it will relax you." – HLT

"Yes, both before and after surgery I did a lot of yoga and meditation. Both helped a lot and I recommend it." – Chris

"I think it helps. You can find lots of different guided meditations and relaxation videos on YouTube for free." – Anonymous

"I started to meditate again after shoulder surgery and I am also reading books. I don't think it helped with the aches and pains, but it made me more accepting. I accepted my shoulder would never be the same. I can't do the things I could do when I was young, and maybe being mindful of who I am has brought me greater peace." – BHW

"I practiced guided imagery with headphones on. There are many programs for dealing with pain and discomfort." – Caroline M.

"Absolutely! Deep breathing and relaxation techniques have been a cornerstone of my recovery." – Madeline

"To be honest wasn't gonna let my doc turn me into a druggie. I meditated every day after surgery. At least it helped me relax. Sometimes, I used Tylenol, but nothing ever stronger." –Anonymous

"I am a firm believer in meditation when I am in pain." – Jackie M.

"I'm practical. Meditation does help, but in the immediate post-op days, you're probably going to need something stronger for pain relief. Meditation can help alleviate the anxiety that can occur when you're in severe pain and I see it as a good adjunct, but if you need medication, use it." – Susanne Q.

"I had a reflexology person do reflexology for my husband and he said it really relaxed him." – Sue

5. Pill Taking

"Make sure you have filled your regular prescriptions ahead of time. You won't feel like trudging off to the drugstore for a while. Obviously, pain pills will come after surgery if you need them." - Anonymous

"Look, there's a chance you're going to be in pain after surgery. You may be prescribed pain medication at regular intervals. I bought a pill organizer with six or eight compartments. Then I set my iPhone alarm at the intervals the doctor prescribed and keeping track was easy." – Richard

"As long as there are no kids in the house, transfer your pills to non-childproof caps before you have surgery. I think your pharmacist will do it for you." – Steve G.

"To be honest I stopped taking pain medication after the second day. I was left with a vial of, I don't know, 30 or more pain pills. I found a service where you can mail

those pills to be destroyed. I didn't want that stuff in the house." – BHW

6. Nausea

"I learned a trick when I visited a relative in a major hospital up in Boston. As I was sitting there talking to him, I was smelling popcorn. At first, I thought I was imagining things but when his nurse came in I asked her about it. She told me the smell of popcorn seems to help patients when they come out of anesthesia to keep them from getting nauseous. Tried it myself after surgery and it calmed me down, or maybe I was just hungry and wanted popcorn! Maybe it will help shoulder surgery patients!" – Harold W.

"For when I felt nauseous after my first shoulder surgery, I kept a supply of chicken broth and applesauce on hand. Both seemed to help settle me down." – Dick C.

7. Cold Therapy

Ice Machine Tips

"Ice may be your best friend like they tell you, but you will go crazy keeping enough ice in the house for your ice machine. Here's what a lot of us do. Before surgery save about eight small plastic bottles. Fill them and freeze them. Put around four at a time in your ice machine then fill to line with water and then just rotate the bottles. A plastic ice bottle will keep frozen for 8-10 hours or more." – Sarah C.

"My ice machine was my best friend, but whenever I used it my whole body felt frozen. I bought a small throw blanket and put it in the dryer to heat it up then wrapped it around [me]. Sounds crazy, but my shoulder stayed nice and cool and the rest of my body was warm." – Jeffrey G.

"I rented one and it was a godsend. I could fall asleep with it on and not have to worry about skin damage or getting up and changing ice packs. The machine also

gives my shoulder a feeling of gentle compression and it feels good." – Ruth W.

"Ice machines have many benefits over ice packs. The ice machine is actively circulating water through a pad you place on the injured area that maintains the water temperature about 42 F. The risk of frostbite is lessened because the pad is on top of a layer or two of clothing. On the other hand, ice packs are much cooler and solid ice. With an ice pack, you can leave it on for maybe 20 minutes at a time." – J.S.

"You can usually find used ice machines on sites like Nextdoor but the problem is to find one with a shoulder wrap attachment. You'll probably have to order one of those from the manufacturer and I found they were about half the price of a new machine. I would not rent a machine in any case." – BHW

"The pain from my rotator cuff surgery has been more intense than the original injury. The ice machine has been amazing. I didn't rent it. I bought it straight out. I've since used it for my plantar fasciitis. It's worth every penny." – Corey

Ice Packs

"Get a muffin pan and place small plastic disposable cups in each well. Fill to about ¾ of a cup of water. Ice will last a lot longer in either ice packs or ice machines" – SW

"I just froze water in quart baggies." – Elaine P.

"You can make homemade gel packs. One cup of 70% rubbing alcohol plus two cups of water in double Ziploc bags and put in freezer until you need them." – Linda

"I never bought an ice machine; my insurance wouldn't pay for it. I am not trying to give you a commercial, but I love my Chattanooga ColPac Ice Packs! I have three of them and keep rotating them." – Charlotte J.

8. Sling Comfort

You might need to wear a sling for up to six weeks or more depending on your procedure. The following tips were offered by patients to ease discomfort on the affected arm and shoulder.

"I took a pair of fuzzy socks, cut out the toe part and put it over my elbow. I would rotate and wash them every other day. It made the sling more comfortable and less itchy." – Fred K.

"Tip for anyone wearing the sling who has pain: I cut the elbow out of mine." – Joe

"Put a hand towel between your arm and the sling." - Anonymous

"I got a seatbelt pad to put over my sling strap. It's lots more comfortable." – Paul W.

"I used a seatbelt cover. It helped ease my shoulder pain after I took off the sling." – Dave

"I have worn long-sleeve cotton t-shirts since day three and I haven't had any skin issues." – Dana W.

"I got hot and itchy where my arm was rubbing against the sling. I used a mentholated body powder and it helped absorb moisture and calmed the itching." – Mike D.

"I cut a fleece baby blanket into quarters. The pieces were the perfect size for my sling. A friend of mine who had surgery cut the legs off toddler pajamas and slid her arm into those inside her sling." – Lisa

"My best advice is if you're still in a sling and get a cold, tighten it up a bit. Stabilize the shoulder joint because coughing and sneezing can cause pain like nobody's business." – Lauri

9. "Shoulder Stations" or Baskets and Carts

I call them "Shoulder Stations." As I live in a small home, I didn't need but one, but they make a lot of sense in a larger home or a multi-level home. The baskets are "hoarding places" where you can keep supplies. With the baskets, you don't have to keep getting up and down to find something. You don't have to go from room to room to get the basics. These are especially helpful in the days following surgery if you have a balance problem or you require a walker.

"Before surgery, I went to the dollar store and bought a few baskets. I placed them in the bedroom, den, bathroom and living room. I put things in each basket like cheap reading glasses, hand lotion, and hand sanitizer. For the one in the bedroom, I put in an eye mask to block out the light, even lavender oil and the television remote. It worked out really well for me." – Perry

"I made up a kitchen basket. I put in paper plates, plastic knives, spoons and forks and napkins. I didn't feel like doing dishes or silverware." – Chris

"I have a small ranch house and when I was alone I went from living room to kitchen to office to bathroom, etc. Sometimes I was really tired from the anesthesia or in a lot of pain and I didn't feel like getting up again. I had a small canvas cart in the shed. I brought it into the house and filled it with snacks, lotion, backscratcher, cell charger, bottled water and other stuff. This way I wheeled my supplies around with me. You can also steal a little wagon from your grandkid!" – Valerie

"I put all of my everyday toiletries in a decorative wicker basket on my bathroom counter, including toothpaste and toothbrush, hair brushes, nail file and scissors, mouthwash, razor, shave cream, skin lotion and medications. It made it easier for me the first few weeks after my shoulder replacement." – Susannah F.

Water (Bottles)

"I would shop around for a great water bottle that you can use one-handed, as the pull tops can be rough." - Anonymous

"I bought a couple of large plastic tumblers with lids and straws." - Anonymous

10. Personal Hygiene

Our fellow "slingers" are not shy about sharing their personal hygiene accomplishments. Days before my own surgery, I remember hearing from a patient who wrote, "I'm so proud of myself — after seven weeks, I wiped my bum with my left hand today!"

Another recently said, "After six weeks of looking like a sheepdog, I put my hair in a ponytail today!"

Personal hygiene is a basic need and all of us share in the necessity of taking care of ourselves. The following personal hygiene tips will prove to be useful. Please note that the words are real, but the identities are altered.

Using the Bathroom

"I highly recommend body/baby wipes in the first days after surgery. You will never feel clean unless you wipe like you are used to doing it." – Carol

"I'll be honest. Before surgery, I was worried about using the bathroom. I was afraid I was not going to be able to wipe after surgery because anything I did with my arm hurt. But surprisingly by the time my bowels were moving, it wasn't an issue. Maybe my surgery wasn't too serious. Just clean yourself as you normally would. Use wipes if you feel you need to." – J.G.

"If you're a guy, it's not always easy to pee while wearing a sling, especially after you've just had surgery and you're wearing trousers and you can only use one hand. It was easier to wear elastic waistbands, pull down the pants and sit!" – Laurence S.

"Cleaning yourself with the non-dominant hand is next to impossible. A nurse friend suggested I get a mustard and ketchup squeeze bottle set and fill one with fresh water and one with soapy water. I used those bottles to clean myself then I wiped. You won't regret practicing before surgery." – Gina B.

"I wore a very loose-fitting gown the first few days. It eliminated the problem of pulling up pants after going to the bathroom. If you have major shoulder surgery, pulling things up is impossible without assistance. You will not be modest after surgery, trust me!" – Marla

"I'm big on hand sanitizer. Let's be honest. You won't be as thorough in your personal hygiene that first couple of weeks. Use hand sanitizer whenever you get the urge." – Richard S.

"They make something called the 'Bottom Buddy.' It's a wipe on a stick to help you clean yourself." – Shirley

"I used an extendable toilet paper wand. There are many different brands and I guess they all work the same. Practice before you have surgery in case you need to do it." – Della

"When I had surgery seven months ago, I ordered a 'Bottom Buddy' for reaching behind to wipe. Don't want to give out too much information, but it's something I really needed and something that worked!" – Charles P.

"In the days right after surgery make sure where you sleep is pretty close to the bathroom. Don't be concerned if you need to urinate more often than usual. At least it's a good idea to be close just to give you comfort."
– Stan M.

Laxatives

"Painkillers plug up your damn insides like cement (lol). It's another reason to hate them. Even before surgery, I started to take in more fibers like Metamucil. I also drank plenty of water. Three days after surgery I was regular." – Jack

"I highly recommend laxatives, laxative teas and prunes, especially if you have been on painkillers. The nurses in the hospital may recommend some things to you as well. Listen to them. Drink plenty of water!"

"Kind of personal, but I stocked up on laxatives, stool softeners, prunes and laxative teas. If you're not on a lot of painkillers, a few days after surgery you will be fine." – Lisa G.

Toilet Fixtures/ Toilet Paper Holder

"When I installed a grab bar in the shower, it was suggested I put a grab bar by the toilet. Due to arthritis, I am unsteady. When I was wearing the sling, the toilet grab bar helped to steady me. It's not easy getting old!" – Phil S.S.

"I used a standing toilet paper holder and I put it on the right side. It was much easier to access." – Jack

11. Showers and Shower Safety
"If you're going to slip and fall, you're going to hit something, most likely the wall or the rim of the tub.

A bar will help steady you as you fall so at least it might be a more controlled fall." – Betty A.

"We all like privacy in the bath, but if you're shy please get over it and get into the habit of keeping the door unlocked. God forbid you fall in the tub after surgery and it's hard to get to you." – Gloria P.

"I have a grab bar and I love it. It was installed in the shower stall wall prior to me buying the house. I also have a shower chair and I use that too." – Norman D.

"I am petrified of falling in the shower — no, make that terrified. I installed a grab bar. They sell them with suction cups. I think it's good for temporary use, but I'm thinking about having my handyman install one on the wall." – JG

"I am still pretty steady on my feet. I did not put in a grab bar in the shower, but I did buy a 'medical height-adjustable bathtub safety rail' to help me get in and out of the tub for showering. I really love my hot baths. When I *felt up to it, I used the rail to raise and lower me into the bathtub. What a luxury!"* – Betty A.

"I have the suction cup type one and have a mat with suction cups on the floor of the tub. By the way, I have a shower caddy with soap and shampoo within easy reach on the wall, not above my head." – Nancy S.

"I have a walk-in shower, but with the rotator cuff and my arthritis I am afraid of slipping, so I put towels on my shower floor. I'd rather have wet floors than a dry broken bone." – Jannette W.

"If you can, have your plumber or handyman replace your existing showerhead with a detachable shower hose. They are easy to use and will help to keep the incision dry. You don't have to spend a fortune for a basic model." – Marla J.

"I recommend you buy a handheld detachable shower head. They make models that attach to the regular shower head with magnets. It is the best way to keep clean all over your body." – Scott R.

Showering, Slings and Other Gadgets

"I had a total shoulder replacement. I know they make mesh arm slings for showering but my doctor never said anything about it. They're only about $12. Still, I got out of the shower, got dressed and put on my regular sling without any problem." – BHW

"I bought a mesh sling on Amazon. Love it! It was a good backup when I wanted to clean my sling or take a break. I think Walgreens and CVS sell them too." – LG

"I didn't buy a mesh sling. It was kind of a waste of money. I just cut the bottom third off a shirt, pulled it up and pinned it and used that to keep my arm from flopping around." – Ford G.

"I was told to let my arm hang and allow water to run over it and that shower slings were a waste of money." – Clive

"I bought a mesh sling and it was worthless. It didn't support the arm and just got in the way. The surgeon's PA told me to just let the arm hang down while I was in the shower." – James

"In the shower, I used a small or partially deflated beach ball and set it slightly higher than my waist. It helped my arm stay in position!" – SM

"My husband had rotator cuff surgery two years ago, and to support his arm and shoulder while taking a shower, he put an empty milk jug under his forearm and held it in place with his thumb through the handle. He's a pretty clever guy!" – Wanda S.

"When my wife was at work the first few days after my surgery, I put a plastic step stool in the bathroom so I didn't have to reach up to adjust the shower head or to get stuff from the top shelf of the cabinet." – Joel K.

Showers/Wound Covering

"I've had a couple of shoulder surgeries and in my case, I had to cover up the incision. By trial and error, I've used Cling Wrap, Glad Press-and-Seal and, while it's not too fashionable (!), trash bags that have been cut down and modified."

"Don't forget large waterproof dressings if you need a dressing change. My husband did my first change with large square ones and the second change he used regular adhesive bandages." – Linda

"I have used Nexcare bandages or press and seal Saran Wrap products for keeping out water while showering" – Mike D.

71

Styling hair can be a problem following shoulder surgery, especially when you have a limited range of motion. There seemed to be consensus that short hair was the best solution. Here are a few hair care tricks and tips that other shoulder surgery patients have tried before you:

"I went back to work after four weeks. My hair dryer stand was a life changer for me. It was like my other arm and allowed me to brush out my hair so that I looked almost normal and not like a drowned rat!" – Donna P.E.

"Love my blow dryer stand. It makes that part of my getting ready all that much easier." – Nancy S.

"When I had shoulder surgery three years ago I purchased a hair dryer stand on Amazon. It has been an absolute lifesaver!!" – Kim S.

"My friend Susan had rotator cuff surgery and she used an electric hair straightening brush which she said did a decent job of helping her to style her hair while she was in a sling. If you have one, it's worth a try." – Gloria L

"Before surgery, I cut my hair pretty short. It was easy to use a hair dryer with my hair that length. By the time it grew back, I was out of a sling." – Shirrele

"Cut your hair short, it will grow back!" – Amanda

"I used a product called 'No Rinse Shampoo' that worked pretty well. I used it for the first week after surgery when I wasn't able to shower. I could do it over the sink and my wife helped me dry it with a towel." – Richard P.

"Don't forget the hair ties or scrunchies. Keep it clean and simple. Make sure you practice with one hand before surgery."

"You're not going to feel like styling your hair in the days after surgery, so why not use a hair turban?" – Totsie

"Seriously? I didn't feel like doing much of anything, especially styling my hair. After a couple of weeks, I had my husband drag me to the hair stylist. I was in Heaven!" – Barb

Getting to the Back!

"Nothing can drive you crazier than an itch you can't reach! Get a telescopic back scratcher if you can. Every little comfort helps." – Marge K.

"Get a back scratcher! Even one of those cheapo ones they sell in those Asian gift shops is better than nothing." – Paul T.

"My back itched a lot following surgery and I found the best way to stop it was to put on lotion. Believe it or not, they make lotion applicators that do a pretty good job of applying lotion to your back." – Kenneth

"I bought an applicator online called an '18-inch, semi-flexible, unbreakable lotion applicator.' When you have one arm in a sling and you're alone with an itch, it's great!" – Carol

"Don't do anything that throws you off balance in the shower. They make all kinds of long-handled brushes, sponges and loofahs. Put soap on them from a pump bottle and then do your back and legs that way." – Doris B.

Personal Grooming/Hygiene Liquids

"Make sure that shampoos, soaps, conditioners and lotions are all pumps. Flip-top containers or any containers that screw off can be tough." – Joseph W.

"I bought spray deodorant today. It's a lifesaver because I still have trouble lifting my arm." – Sam W.

"They make spray deodorant that is easier to apply than stick deodorants." – Larry W.

Shaving

"There are companies that make razors with shaving cream inside of them. If you're immobilized, it lets you put on shaving cream with one hand and then shave."
– Peter G.

"Buy a travel size can of aerosol shave cream or shave gel. They are smaller and easier to handle than a larger size. In fact, I used all kinds of travel sizes during my recovery, including deodorants." – BHW

"Ladies, they make a long-handled razor for shaving your legs when you are pregnant. I tried it with one arm following my rotator cuff [surgery] because it seemed like a good idea. I would say it worked 'fair.' Use it if you're going out fancy and need to wear a dress. For the most part, wear long pants until after a month or two." –
Gina A.

"I wound up dusting off my old Norelco and shaved with that until eight weeks post-surgery. My alternative was to grow a beard and I hate them! I didn't feel like messing around with razors and shaving cream." – Robert F.

Dental Hygiene

"I used dental picks rather than dental floss or tape. They make a few different kinds. By the way, when you open the package put them inside a Ziploc bag and that way you won't have dental picks all over the floor." – Robbie B.

"I like toothpaste that comes in flip-top containers that you can squeeze out onto a toothbrush [so] you don't have to worry about a twist-off cap." – Mark

"I used a Waterpik as I found it did a really good job." – Ephraim

"There are a few companies that make travel toothbrushes that are fairly good. They have the toothpaste

built into the handle. I used a Colgate that had disposable travel brushes with 24 in a pack. There were other companies and you can find them on Amazon. Of course, a travel toothbrush can last a few days at least." – Carol B.

12. Clothing

Prior to writing *The Friendly Handbook of Shoulder Surgery Coping Tips and Tricks*, I had no idea which topic would create the most interest and funny stories among those recovering from shoulder surgeries. Little did I know that clothing would be the subject that generated the most comments.

I have logically divided the comments between women's clothing and men's clothing, but even that division can be a little "artificial." For example, many women liked to wear men's shirts such as Dickies work shirts! My suggestion is that you read through all of the comments and pick out those that strike an interest. In general, I would say that over the first six weeks or so, most patients dress for function, not high fashion.

After surgery, many people reported that their skin was sensitive, dry and itchy.

If certain types of fabrics bothered you before surgery, chances are you will be bothered even more for a month or two after. Be careful of a bargain if the fabric is normally bothersome to you.

Women's Clothing

Of all of the articles of women's clothing, and of all of the comments, "The Bra" created the most controversy. There were almost as many thoughts as female patients. Here then are comments, tips and tricks that may be of help.

My thanks to the women who were kind enough to help me decipher the language of women's underwear!

"If you can, try a tankini bathing suit top in place of the bra. You can step into it and just pull it up." – Joanne P.

"I wore and still wear (after many months) a camisole instead of a bra." – Jane

"I used tank tops that already came with a built-in bra. It was a good solution for me." – Bess N.

"I use bralettes that I buy at Walmart, but many stores sell them. You can also buy them online. They are easy to wear and the straps miss my incision. There's no pressure on my scar." – Betty P.

"In the first weeks, when I went out I found a strapless bra to be the best option. I did it up in the front and then turned it around one-handed. For just around the house, I had an idea for making my own bra. I modified a bra in a tank top by cutting one strap and using Velcro. It's good to be creative." – O.R.

"I was able to get into my bra pretty quickly. I hooked the bra then loosened the straps to be as loose as possible. I put on my bra from the floor up. I put my feet in first and then worked it up against my body. First I put [the] strap on my surgical arm then the other arm." – Ginny

"After surgery, I used the same type of bra as always: no straps over the shoulder. I used tape that sticks to the skin to keep the front secure and in place. I have never hooked a bra in the back and now, with my rotator cuff, I couldn't do it. It is natural for me to hook it in the front and turn it around." – Sheila M.

"I'm large and I can't just flop around! I tried three different styles. One couldn't work at all, the second might be good for going back to work down the road in a couple months, but for the near future, the one I liked the most was front-closing.

The best part was that the straps use Velcro so I can undo one if it's irritating my incisions or I just need a break. You can easily find them online." – Glenda M.

"I use a front-hook, T-back bra. The straps miss the incision completely and that's the best possible outcome."
– Carol M.

"Victoria's Secret makes a front-zip sports bra that is very comfortable and functional." – Gale E.

"I use a front-closure racerback bra. Since [it is a] racerback, the strap doesn't sit on my incision." – N.D.O.

"I found that a bra tube was best for me in the months after surgery." – Jennifer S.

"I have worn front-closing racerbacks ever since my shoulder surgeries a few months ago." – Mary

"I used a microfiber bra that is easy to get on and off with minimal arm movement. I recommend you buy them larger than normal, maybe an extra size." – Gale B.

"Hubby took me shopping. Got a set of three bras from Walmart for $10. They were a size larger than my usual exercise bras. Easy to get in and strap by the neck. So far not bad." – Anonymous

"I went strapless or I just didn't put a strap on my shoulder for about two months or so." – Anonymous

"I wore camis at first, then I wore stretchy, cheap sports bras for a while." – Dale

"A bra was the most difficult item for me to put on. I had to purchase a bra that fastened in the front and I didn't put a shoulder strap on. I loosened it all the way and let it dangle — I also had assistance with that." – Marla

"Got a sports bra today that goes up by the neck. It's not too bad." – Pat D.

"In the beginning, I wore a strapless tube bra. I'd wiggle in feet first. Later on, I got a tank-top bra and I wiggled in the same way, but because of my incision, I only wore one strap. It wasn't easy." – Phyllis M.

83

"My absolute recommendation is front-closure bras. Go buy some. Anything else is just too difficult when you're healing." – Margaret

Bras, discomfort

"Had rotator cuff surgery. After seven weeks and one day, I tried a real bra. Was not ready for that yet! The pressure of the strap across the repair is what did me in! I went back to [a] stretchy T-back option." – JR

"My advice? Forget underwear and bras for a while! Wear loose, wide-neck tops or loose, front-button tops and loose, elastic-waist pants for around the house. After surgery, you're not going to be in the mood to go to a fancy restaurant."

"It took me months to be able to put on and wear a real bra. Don't rush it." – ME

"Between the sling and the thick Dickies work shirts that I wore, no one realized I was not wearing a bra. The pain of the straps was just too much to handle." – Arlene W.

"In the weeks following surgery, I couldn't wear a bra. I used large men's t-shirts and ponchos that I crocheted. Anything else was just too painful." – Mary

"No bra for me the first weeks. I used t-shirts, baggy sweaters and ponchos. You won't be able to reach behind you or stand the pain of straps bearing down on your shoulder in any case. Even sports bras can be tough because you have to use an upward motion to put them on." – Shirley A.

"It took me months before I was able to wear a bra. Enjoy it while it lasts!" – Dana W.

"It was well over two months after shoulder surgery 'til I could walk in my home and not want to rip it [the bra] off right away." – Julia

"It's been eight weeks and I'm not there yet (for my regular bra). I wear a super stretchy, thin-strap T-back." – Erynn

"I just could not stand wearing a bra strap on my shoulder. It's six months post-op and I am still not back into a regular bra. It's the straps, I can't stand the pressure." – SS

"A friend of mine had some success with silicone strap cushions about two months after her shoulder surgery. They can take a little of the pressure off the shoulders while you're getting used to wearing a bra again. They didn't work for me, to be honest, but they helped her." – Kelly

Shirts and Blouses – Women

The women who commented on "shirts and blouses," and in fact all clothing, were practical and stylish at the same time.

While form and function were more important than fashion, the solutions struck me as being quite clever and stylish. The following tips and tricks might put you more at ease as to what to wear after shoulder surgery.

"I came up with an idea I might turn into a business. I took a t-shirt and cut it along each side and under the arms, then I put in Velcro along the sides. I messed up the first one, but the second turned out pretty good! As an undershirt, it worked very well." – Linda A.

"I'm a big believer in stretchy tops from stores like Walmart and Target. Goodwill is another place to get loose shirts. Don't waste your money on good stuff. I have been through different shoulder surgeries in all seasons and made do." – Kathy K.

"I liked loose, oversized shirts with a big neck. Put your 'bad arm' in first, then over [your] head and then the good arm. I liked t-shirts rather than button shirts as I found the buttons challenging." – Frieda

87

"I found some cheap, warm and super stretchy long-sleeve shirts on sale at Walmart. They were easy to get on and off. I also bought V-neck super stretch shirts and some velour sweater knits. You can be comfortable and look nice without spending a fortune." – Margarete O.

"In the weeks following surgery, I wore a lot of V-neck cotton t's so to put those on, I bent over toward floor, let my surgical arm dangle, slipped that arm in first and then gently pulled the shirt up over my head and good arm, so I slipped the good arm in last." – Marla

"I lived in tank tops and oversized, button-up shirts for the first five weeks. I am just now able to wear a sweatshirt and a vest as a jacket." – Susie

"If you don't mind rocking your battle scars (and why would you?), after surgery I started wearing an 'off the shoulder' short-sleeve blouse and 'tunic tops' that I found on Amazon.

They were lightweight and flowy, fairly attractive and hardly put any weight on the incision." – Jenni G.

"Go to Goodwill and buy some big loose, button-up men's shirts. If you're worried about where they came from(!), take them to the dry cleaners and get them laundered the first time around. They look good with leggings too." – Leslie

"I bought women's long 'kimono sleeve' loose-fit tunics. They worked well with flowy cardigans." – Anonymous

"On Amazon, I found what they called 'kimono loose-fit tunics'. Several companies sell them. I bought a set of three of them. They are stretchy enough to put on and to take off with one arm. You put them on by putting your bad (surgically repaired) arm in first, then your head through the hole, then your good arm, then pull down. I wore these constantly for the first three weeks. They look great with sweatpants, yoga pants or leggings.

I'm not saying you can dress like a fashion model after surgery, but it's not difficult to look good." – Joanne R.

"I love my kaftans! They come in a million different colors and are easy to put on so you can look dressy for not too much money. Of course, the sling kind of dresses them down, but it makes for great dinner conversation." – Peg

"I like big lady elastic skirts, elastic-waist long skirts and slips. I wore them with oversized flannel shirts and ponchos. I guess it was the old 'Annie Hall' look, but it worked just fine for me!" – Kathie N.

Dresses

"I wore loose dresses for the first two weeks as they were comfortable over my incision. They also helped at toilet time. I am 60, so when I gotta go, I gotta go!" – Catherine P.

"Dresses are awesome after surgery because no one ever warns you about the pants. I'm a huge fan of wearing jeans and unfortunately, I can't even button them after three weeks." – Emilie

"I couldn't put that much pressure on my arm and shoulder after surgery, so I definitely recommend investing in leggings and a dress to go over them." – A.R.

Over-garments – Women

"I really like ponchos, they go over the sling and everything. In warmer weather, wraps and scarves work just fine. Ponchos are very easy to find online as [is] poncho-type rain-gear." – Ingrid

"About a month before I was scoped, we went down to Mexico on vacation. It was right around springtime. Anyway, I brought back a serape. It made for quite a scene, but it worked perfectly. Don't overthink this stuff!" – Amanda V.

"Usually I wore no coat or a light coat if the temperature was close to zero. To be honest I tried to put my poncho on over my sling and it was a pain to get everything 'settled' the way I wanted it to be. The supermarket had a sale on small plush throw blankets. I bought a nice gray one for $2.50 on sale, wrapped it around and used a decorative pin to keep it together. You know, it was perfect." – Sharon

"I had a lightweight but warm quilt jacket. After about two weeks, I would put the jacket on, and then put the sling on. It kept me warm, and in places like the grocery store it 'warned' people to keep clear of my shoulder." – Margaret W.

"I bought a nice down vest online and I wore it over a loose sweater. For most of the winter, I was fine walking around outside." – Sheila M.

"Definitely a vest instead of a jacket." – FNA

Sweaters, Women's

"Look for sales before surgery at stores that carry big soft cheap sweaters. The ones I found were easy on and easy off and only about $8 and adorable." – SW

"I'm a fan of V-neck sweaters because they have a big opening. Just make sure you get one that's a little too large and a plusher material. Bend over, put the surgical arm in first, then your head and finally the good arm." – Joyce S.

Sweatpants

"I bought sweatpants with a normal leg. They're cheap and I don't feel like I'm walking around in pajamas. I hate that feeling." – Monica N.

"There's new materials they use in sweatpants that keep you really toasty in the fall and winter. I bought two pairs at Costco. I wore yoga pants before surgery but I don't recommend them if you've had rotator cuff repair.

They're too difficult to hike up. I would wait a couple of months before trying to put them on." – Jenn P.

Men's Clothing

Slacks and Trousers

"When I first came home from the hospital I couldn't even think about putting on pants other than sweatpants with elastic waistbands. They are comfortable, look OK and [are] cheap. I recommend you go out and buy a few pairs. When you start to feel a little better, you can use the sweatpants for working out." – Russell O.

"Stay away from skinny jeans. They're too hard to put on and take off, and tough to button and zip. Not worth it." – Ken S.

"During the first week or so, I just used drawstring pants so I didn't have to negotiate with zippers, belts and such. I found really cheap pants in Walgreens drugstore, believe it or not." – Tyrone G.

"Belts are tough because until you have gone through months of physical therapy it will be hard for you to reach behind your back. Sit in a chair, put the belt through the loops first, then hike up the pants, then tighten the buckle."
– Larry W.

Shirts – Men

"It's not that hard to wear regular clothing after a total shoulder replacement but the key is to keep the shirts loose. If you are used to a tailored look, get regular-sized shirts. Personally, for those first few weeks, I got my shirts at the thrift shop or I went to the 70%-off rack at Target!"
– Ken B.

"For me so far, button-up flannel shirts have worked great. [They] also protect my arm from a scratchy sling." – Pat

"I just used button-up shirts, nothing form-fitting! Had to learn to put the buttons through the holes with 'mostly' one hand." – Doug Z.

"There are several brands of what I call 'shoulder surgery clothes.' They work with Velcro so you can put them on while wearing a sling. I'm not knocking them. They're clever and fill a need. If you have the money or a good insurance flex plan, go for it. I found that baggy, button-up shirts worked just fine for me. T-shirts a size up worked great too." – Harold W.

"After a week post-surgery, there was no way I could reach around to tuck in my dress shirt. My wife had to do it for me. I couldn't bring her to work with me! As a friend told me, 'Who cares? Let it all hang out.' Now, about five weeks after surgery, I can start to do it but the motion still causes me some pain." – Sam A.

"Tailored shirts are overrated. By that I mean, after total replacement surgery, you want ease and comfort. I bought baggier shirts. I was able to button up the shirts myself after a couple of days. The cuffs took a little longer, maybe a week or so.

Anyway, to put the shirt on, I bent down and put the surgical arm through first, got the shirt around and the other arm was easy." – Stuart L.

"*I'm not exactly a tailor but let me tell you what I did. I bought cheap t-shirts and then I cut them up the side from waist to sleeve. I bought Velcro strips and glued them along the seams. It worked like a charm. When I was finally out of the sling, I chucked the shirts. I then bought three baggy cotton shirts at Walmart for not much more than $10. By the way, the Velcro was about $4, the cloth glue was about $3. [My] comfort was priceless.*" – Gregory G.

Hoodies, Men's

"*After surgery, I was able to get a hoodie on right away with my wife's help. She made a vertical cut on the front side of the 'head hole,' about 4 – 5 inches in length, and made it easier to get on and off. She had me bend forward, let my arms hang and she had me put the surgical arm in first, then the head, then the good arm. You can either buy cheap new hoodies or you can go to places like Goodwill and get them used and really cheap. Just wash the hell out of them. Who cares what they say, you just want function!"* – Bob C.

"I really like hoodies with zippers down the front. They're not too expensive and they last a long time. Buy them a size larger than you need and that way if you're wearing a sling they can go over the sling." – Bob Z.

Sweaters, Men's

"V-neck sweaters were the way to go. You can put them on over a baggy shirt or a t-shirt and it looks pretty good." – Dan

Shoes, Women's and Men's

"It was about two weeks after total shoulder replacement [that] I was able to tie my own sneakers. Prior to that, I bought a pair of shoes with Velcro straps. Style-wise they were clunky, but they were easy to put on and pretty comfortable to wear." – David E.

"Those first weeks after surgery the weather was still pretty nice. I wore sandals and flip-flops and I was pretty much set." – Emily M.

"I wore slip-on shoes for months, especially when it was snowing." – Sam A.

"Here's my recommendations for shoes: boots, slippers, sandals and slip-on shoes with a shoehorn. I didn't tie shoes for a month." – Sandy

"Get a long shoehorn, especially for boots and loafers." – Sandi

"The first three weeks I wore loafers without using socks. They make a gadget to help you put on socks. It's like a plastic sleeve that the socks go over and two cords to pull it up. The problem is that most people need two good hands and pain-free shoulders to use it." – Paul

"I thought the Yaktrax product was clever. They are removable 'cleats' you can put on and take off the bottom of shoes to help you walk in snow or ice. The very last thing

you want to do with a shoulder repair is to fall. Please be super careful on ice." – Annie I.

"My solution to tie-up shoes was pretty simple for a while. I tied them before I had surgery on my rotator cuff. Using a shoe horn, I kind of slipped into them. The bows held pretty well for a few weeks." – Stephen N.

"Have you ever heard of curly shoelaces? Look them up on the internet. They're really clever and let you wear shoes without bending down to tie bows. I just love them. It's worth it to put them in a couple pairs of shoes before shoulder surgery." – Susan

"Everyone seems to have a shoehorn somewhere in the house. Make your life easier and get one with a long handle." – Richard G.

"No high heels for me for several months. No, no, no!" – Judy W.

"It was hard for me to reach down and to tie my shoes after rotator cuff repair. So I sat in a comfy chair, brought my foot up to my chest and tied it like that. It was much easier with slip-ons!" – Pat B.

13. Furniture

While you don't have to spend a fortune on furniture to help you with your recovery, there are a few items to consider that can help you in those first weeks, especially if you work from home. The following furniture items were suggested by patients recovering from shoulder surgery:

"I enjoyed using what they call a bed desk. I propped myself up in bed with several pillows and then put my laptop on top of the bed desk. If I felt like dozing off, I could just put the bed desk aside." – Barbara

"Devote a small bookcase or shelf to a lot of supplies, especially next to your recliner or bed. Just make sure it's against the wall.

I used a small three-shelf bookcase for my ice machine, lotion, remote and stuff like that. Go to a garage sale, don't spend a fortune on it." – Fran O.

"I got my left knee done 18 months ago, and a total shoulder in October. I love my cooking so I bought a 'medical kitchen stool.' It's got an adjustable height, rails and a solid seat back. The seat is set at an angle. Stay away from those chairs on rollers. I think they're dangerous." – Stephen N.

"The reclining bleacher chair was something my son-in-law found for me online. It is a padded bleacher chain that can recline and it even has a pouch on the side for bottled water. It works well on my couch to give my shoulder a better angle. They are inexpensive and come in all types of adjustable sizes." – Jamie Y.

"You can go to almost any garage sale in America and find a TV tray table! The last thing you want to do is have a plate of spaghetti land in your lap!" – John C.

14. "The Gourmet Shoulder Patient Chef"

Maybe you're a highly trained French chef, or perhaps your idea of high-quality food is anything that comes in a can. I guess most of us are somewhere in between. In any case, you will quickly find that preparing and cooking food one-handed presents us with a whole new set of challenges. The following ideas, tips and tricks might help you on your journey from sling to wellness.

Cooking Safety

There are many rules for safety in the kitchen and they are easily found on numerous websites. It is useful to revisit them. Though you may be Julia Child, Gordon Ramsay, Paula Deen, Bobby Flay and Jamie Oliver rolled into one, when you go from two arms and two shoulders down to mostly one, *everything* changes.

I have compiled the top 7 safety high points that appear on almost every cooking safety list. I found it useful to review these rules after I returned from the hospital in a sling.

1. **FIRE!** Got your attention? Watch your sling around the stove whether gas flame, electric or — if you should decide to try it — BBQ. And speaking of heat, always use potholders.

2. Don't be distracted by your company, music, the television, dogs or cats, and don't try to speed through the food preparation. Please, focus on the kitchen task at hand.

3. Knife safety. Be careful and watch how you are holding the knife and cutting. Your "sling hand" will not be straight and steady as usual, especially if it is your non-dominant arm. If the knife slips from your hand, let it fall; don't try to grab it.

4. Wear shoes that will not slip on the kitchen floor. Try to avoid food preparation in bare feet, socks, flip-flops or slick slippers.

5. Anything spilled needs to be immediately cleaned up, especially oils, ice water and small grains such as rice and barley.

6. Do NOT lift anything that is too heavy for you. Wait for help.

7. If you have purchased a new kitchen utensil or piece of equipment, get familiar with it before your surgery, or have someone watch you use it after surgery.

Boiling Water & Other Liquids

"If you've just had surgery, the last thing you want to do if you're alone is to boil water in a big kettle. I like one-cup immersion water boilers. They're very lightweight. [They] unplug easily and best of all, they're fast!" – Iris A.

"Be careful around any kind of boiling water. If boiling water splashes on your sling, it can burn right through onto your arm. If you accidentally drop a kettle or even a cup filled with boiled water, which is what I did, expect painful burns and blisters." – Juli G.

"Watch it around soups, stews and spaghetti sauces. Stir foods away from your body. Keep your distance. Don't lift any heavy pots with one hand." – Betty

Cooking, Food and Wine Tips
"Betty's List of One-Handed Appliances"

A friend of mine (Betty) is a chef with a good sense of humor — just don't try to talk to her while she's busy in the kitchen! Betty has most every kitchen gadget ever created, new and antique. Some people collect baseball cards, others collect postage stamps. Betty buys unusual kitchen gadgets. She heard about my shoulder surgery recovery project, saw me in a sling and came up with a list of appliances and gadgets she felt would be of benefit.

106

I am pleased to include her list and comments in this section. Several of these one-handed gadgets were completely new to me. Every one of them can be purchased online or at retail outlets specializing in kitchenware.

a. *Battery operated pepper mills – These can also be used for sea salt.*

b. *Hand blenders – They're much easier to use than a full-size mixer.*

c. *Paring boards – Sometimes they're also called Swedish cutting boards. They're very clever. They let you cut things with one hand and you can change the positions of the pins to accommodate what you want to cut.*

d. *Baby food processors – They make miniature food processors and blenders that can be handled with one hand.*

e. *Citrus sectioning tools* – *One-handed tools to help you cut large oranges and grapefruits into sections.*

f. *"Solo Grip"* – *One-handed jar opener. It's plastic and you jam the jar into it and can twist off the screw-top cap with one hand.*

g. *Saucepan Stirrer* – *Come in several variations, either over the pot or in the pot, but the best news is that they are hands-free.*

h. *Jar-lid popper* – *Very clever gadget to pop the top of a glass jar one-handed.*

i. *Adjustable food and vegetable slicer*

j. *Banana slicer* – *I saved the best for last! My fave! They make a banana cutter in the shape of a banana. You peel the banana set it in place and it gives you perfect slices.*

"The day before surgery I set up my counter. I put my food processor on the counter along with a few pans. I could slide them over to the stove or sink as needed." – SB

"In the first week, 10 days or so, I always kept a pair of sharp scissors at hand. I couldn't open plastic bags with one hand and I didn't want to risk anything after the cuff repair." – Sandra

"Always keep a sharpened pair of scissors handy to cut plastic bags with vegetables, snack foods and cereals. Let me emphasize the word 'sharp!'" – Andy D.

"After my total shoulder replacement surgery, it hurt my repaired shoulder to cut things, especially Italian bread. This occurred when I held the bread with one hand and sawed back and forth with the other. I got out two wooden cutting boards and staggered one board over the

other with the bread in between. I gently pressed down on the top board and was able to easily cut." – Harold W.

"*I tried an electric knife and personally I didn't like it. It's not as easy as it sounds, you can't control it all that well and I was afraid of the sawing action while cutting.*" – Marvin S.

"*If there is a drawer just underneath the countertop, open the drawer, put the jar inside the drawer and push the drawer closed with your hip, and then take your good hand and open the jar. Just make sure it's a plastic jar!*" – Greta Z.

"*If it's a plastic jar or soda bottle, I just push it against the counter with my hip and unscrew it with my good hand.*" – Carl T.

"*Sit down and squeeze the bottle or jar between your thighs and unscrew lid with a good hand screw. It's like the thigh master!*" – MG

110

"I finally got an electric can opener after my surgery. In addition to my rotator cuff procedure, they had previously removed a joint in my hand due to arthritis. It was painful and difficult to open jars." – BSC

"If you don't want an expensive electric gadget, they do make a one-handed mechanical can opener that works pretty well, and I think it's under ten bucks on Amazon." – Ben

"Before my total shoulder replacement surgery, I decided to get an electric jar opener because I still have problems opening things. It's not going to get better as I age." – John G.

"We bought an electric wine opener for about $20. You just set it on top of the bottle and press the button, then release the cork by pressing another button and Voila! It comes with a charging station." – John S.

"Want to open a bottle of sparkling wine or champagne? Buy some rubber gloves. Remember, don't twist the cork, twist the bottle!" – Jannette W.

"Lots of wines now come in screw-top bottles and I've been told they taste as good as wine with corks. Anyway, it works for me!" – Morris T.

Easy to Prepare Meals/Snack Ideas

"I had friends who went through shoulder surgery before I did and so I knew to have tons of foods prepared well ahead of time. I made soups and froze them as well as stews, spaghetti sauce, clam sauce and lasagna. It didn't make the pain go away, but it tasted good!" – Jen D.

"Any kinds of foods or ready to eat meals you can eat or prepare one-handed! Grapes were nice to snack on, TV dinners, soups with easy-open lids, Jell-O [and] pudding cups were great."

"I have a little wicker basket at hand and I set it up with snack foods in Ziploc bags for during the day when I was alone. This method seemed to work the best because food packaging can be difficult to open." – SB

"Before you go in for surgery, stock up on all condiments that come in squeeze bottles including ketchup, mustard, mayonnaise, honey and even salad dressings."

"Like peanut butter and jelly sandwiches? Peanut butter and jelly come in squeeze bottles." – Hillary

"Ice cream or sherbet in any form, but especially on sticks. Both are great to coat your stomach before you take medications."

"My 5 and 7-year-old nieces were my inspiration. They have all kinds of products that are in tubes including yogurt and peanut butter. They are easy to eat and make great snack foods." – Bruce T.

"Bite-sized fruit is good and helps you avoid constipation after surgery. It doesn't just have to be prunes or dried apricots. Any kind of berry is good — strawberries, blackberries, blueberries, raspberries and such. Apples and pears can be messy. They are not so easy to cut up either. Apple and pear slicers generally require two hands. It takes more pressure than you think to push down on the fruit." – Eric P.

"Bite-sized veggies are great. You can get washed and peeled baby carrots, pre-cut cauliflower and broccoli florets, cherry tomatoes, green onions, radishes and even pre-cut mixed greens."

"Single-portion cereals such as instant oatmeal can be good, providing you have easy access to a microwave."

"I made some crock-pot stews and put them in the freezer."

"Chips and salsa or chips and hummus are old standbys, but the combos are messy as hell if you're down to one arm. I suggest you get someone to subdivide the chips into Ziploc bags beforehand. They also sell small portions of Queso dips, hummus, and salsa to make life easier."

"Single-serve protein drinks are manageable. While they also make single serve cheese wedges and baby Gouda type cheeses, they can be messy unless you get a little help."

15. Traveling
Going through TSA Screening

"I'm 12 weeks post-op for my total shoulder replacement surgery and I still can't get my arm high enough to go through a scanner. I need to work on that for my next flight. If I need to go somewhere in an emergency, I've got to tell the TSA agent." – Bill D.

"I wondered if my shoulder hardware would set off the scanner. Sure enough, three days before a trip I had to report to jury duty. They had a scanner at the courthouse and it immediately picked up on my new shoulder." – Steve K.

In-Flight

"Where will you sit? First of all, if you're wearing a sling, some airlines will let you pre-board so you can find a comfortable spot. My personal rule of thumb is bulkhead. If you're in a sling they won't want you in an emergency row. Stay away from all the middle seats. The aisle seat is good and bad. In flight, you're generally OK but when people get on or off it's a guarantee you're going to get bumped. I like the window seat, to be honest." – Charlie P.

"I traveled two months post-surgery, about a two-and-a-half-hour flight. I didn't need a sling at that point, but I wore it so other people knew I was injured. It is sort

of an insurance policy to protect you from other people

slamming doors on you and such." – Kris

Walking the Dog

"Oh, do I have a story. Today I decided to take my

Jack Russell Terrier for a walk because I figured my

rotator cuff repair was well on its way to healing. Wow, he

pulled me across the driveway. I don't think I can

remember such pain. How stupid I was. You can bet he

went back in the house on his own. LOL." – Betty B.

"My dogs have always been my walking buddies,

and I started walking them again two weeks after surgery.

My surgical shoulder (arm) has never touched the leash. It

may be many more months. At first, I would take them one

at a time. This week for the first time I took them both, but

you have to be extremely careful. They are trained to heel,

but you still have to be careful." – Alanna G.

"I use a European leather leash [note: there are many variations of this leash in nylon] *with my dogs that wraps around my waist like a belt and hooks to the dog's collar. Greatest leash ever. Trainers say these leashes are better to walk with regardless of whether you have an injury or not because you're not sending vibes down the leash so your dog is more comfortable on walks."* – Phil M.

"Unless you have a well-trained dog, I mean a 'wonder dog,' things can go south in a heartbeat. I work with dogs, teaching many competitive agility classes a week. When a dog lunges at another dog or a cat or squirrel, you're going to reach out without thinking about your bad arm. I learned my lesson and it almost cost me another shoulder operation. If you have had a shoulder procedure, find a leash that will keep you safe." – Pamela K.

16. Your Home

We often look at things too closely, without seeing the big picture. With an arm in a sling, life changes for all of us. We should step back and take a careful look around our environment.

For example, if we normally enter a home through a front door, but the front door has steps leading to it, or if those steps "twist" or if those steps can get coated with ice in the winter, are we better off entering through a side entrance?

Where should we sleep? While we normally sleep in a bedroom, suppose the bedroom is on another floor, or might be too small to accommodate a recliner (if we need one) or is filled with tripping hazards — are we better off setting up shop in another area of the home?

The bathroom needs to be within an easy distance from where we sleep, and the bathroom needs to be safe. In talking with many people who have had shoulder surgeries,

119

it is very wise to have someone you trust to go through your home with you *weeks before* you have shoulder surgery.

Are some of the doors and hallways too narrow or dangerous? Are the windows difficult to open with one arm? Are any of the possible exits to the home, no matter the size of the home, hard to navigate?

Is the kitchen safe or are some of the fixtures, cabinets, and drawers difficult to open?

We all enter shoulder surgery with a different set of medical conditions. Your particular kind of shoulder surgery might be quite simple and straightforward and you may have no other pre-existing medical conditions. However, others might have had hip and knee replacements, or perhaps they have severe arthritis or require a walker or cane or any other number of conditions. When going through the home, view the situation in terms of the patient's condition.

I know all of this sounds overly simple but you might be surprised at how many well-meaning friends who volunteer to go on a walk-through with you through your home completely forget you might have a bad knee in addition to an arm in a sling. It can make a big difference as to where you "set up shop" when you come home from the surgical center or hospital.

Home Safety Tips for Slingers
Sweeping

"Sweeping my floors is hard with one hand. I did figure out that I could use my foot to keep the dustpan in place." – Paula A.

"My kids bought me a 'Roomba' robot vacuum. I love my kids!" – Sheryll P.

Floors

"My wife usually assigns me floor cleaning on our cleaning days, but with my sling and recent surgery, I got off for good behavior. The floors were just too slippery." – Sandy

"I need to warn everyone about those small rag rugs on any kind of wood floor. I stepped off of one and went flying. By the Grace of all that's Holy, I landed on the couch. All I could think of was a return to surgery." – John F.

Spare Keys

"I put a spare key in an empty flowerpot on my porch. During the day when my wife was at work, I was afraid of what would happen if I fell down while I was in a sling. I didn't want to leave the doors unlocked. I wanted to make sure the firemen could get in." – Cal M.

Smoke Alarms/Fire

"The last thing you want to do — or can do with a sling on — is to put batteries in the smoke detector. Make sure you do this before surgery. Same with carbon monoxide detectors." – BHW

"If you live alone or if you're at home alone always think about fire safety. This is important if you're in a sling. What's the best exit? Are the escape routes filled with junk? Are any doors blocked? Think all this stuff through." – Peter B.

"When was the last time you checked your fire extinguisher and do you even have one? If not, get one!" – Shirley G.

Reaching for Things around the Home

"I don't recommend reaching for things. It strains your good arm and can throw you off balance. It is also a good way to get clunked on the head. I liked standing on a stool or step stool and in that way, I was closer to the same level." – Bart E.

"Get a very sturdy step stool with side guard rails and never attempt to reach up for things with your arm in a sling. Get up to the level of the shelf or whatever." – Bob H.

"Grabber tools are the way to go. The older I get and the more arthritic I become, the more my grabber comes in handy. When I needed surgery on my rotator cuff [it was] a life-saver. They are pretty cheap and come in a couple different sizes." – Susan C.

"Grabbers are OK for picking things off the floor but be careful if you're going after a can of peas or something on a top shelf. It's an easy way to get clunked on the head. Guys who used to use them in those little old-fashioned grocery stores had two good hands. They'd catch things on the way down." – Siggie M.

17. Driving

There were responses to my questionnaire where people said they were driving "immediately" after surgery and they boasted, "Well, no one told me I couldn't!"

Sorry friend, that excuse won't hold up in court, especially if you are the driver at fault.

During those first several weeks when you must wear a sling, please use carpools, public transportation, Uber, Lyft and taxis, or please ask spouses and friends to take you where you need to go. Even after the sling comes off, it may be a few weeks before you have the strength to control the wheel. Power steering doesn't mean effortless steering.

"Finally drove at seven and a half weeks. I had my arm in a sling with a bolster for six and a half weeks then needed to build back my strength and confidence to where I could control the vehicle in case of an emergency." – Cal M.

"To me, driving with a sling is a lot like people who drive drunk. If you hit ice or snow, you can't steer your car. My uncle is a cop. He told me every state has laws against driving one-handed without controls." – Barry M.

"My surgeon said she was happy for me to drive after four weeks post-op with a shoulder replacement. My

physical therapist absolutely disagreed and said he would not be happy until I went for eight weeks before driving. He told me when I first felt comfortable to go around the block that I should do it after nine weeks! I drive a manual and the operated arm is the gear-shift arm, so it was a few months before I felt fully comfortable driving." – Fred

"*My surgeon said I could drive with a sling as long as I was no longer taking strong meds. As it turned out, the cushion sling was cumbersome. I waited more than a month before I felt comfortable behind the wheel.*" – Carl

"*Don't drive until sometime after they tell you. I drove sometime after I got the sling off at five weeks.*" – Dennis

"*I was warned not to drive until I was done with my sling. I have three weeks to go. If I got into an accident, even if it wasn't my fault, or I got pulled over and they saw my condition, it would not be good. It's not worth the risk to me.*" – Anonymous

"My first post-op exam is tomorrow. My doc said no driving for six weeks. I have to wear a sling with an abduction pillow for four weeks and then the sling alone for at least another two depending on my progress. I really, really want to drive. I am the only driver in my household as my husband is disabled. It's terrible depending on other people, but I just don't have the strength." – Thelma

"Yeah, I cheated. I drove with the sling on. I should have known better. It was not safe. I overcompensated on the ice with the one arm and almost went up on the curb. I was lucky and stupid." – John T.

18. Odds 'n Ends!

The following are additional items that those (or their relatives) who have had rotator cuff surgery or shoulder replacement surgery found helpful. These were mentioned just once, but they deserve their own category because they may also help you in your recovery.

- Electronic lap blanket – *"They make a small electric blanket that can be used as a lap blanket or a shawl. I had surgery in December and my body was always too hot or too cold. I used the lap blanket all the time, especially when I was using the ice machine on my shoulder."* – Beth I.

- Fan Pull – *"I extended the chain fan pull by about a foot so I wouldn't have to reach up and try to grab it. I put a decorative pull thingy at the end."* – Daniel T.

- Flashlight – *"I kept two flashlights. One was a plug-in not far from where I was sleeping and [the other was] a powerful battery-operated flashlight that I kept on the nightstand."* – Ben

- Batteries – *"Don't forget new batteries for the TV remote or the remote on your garage door opener."* – Anonymous

- Steering Assist Knob – *"I found several steering assist knobs online. They can help you turn the steering wheel with one arm."* – Elaine (Note: Please check the legality of this item in your state).

- Velcro – *"It's always good to have extra Velcro around the house, especially if you want to modify a t-shirt."* – Tracey M.

- Empty squeeze bottles – *"I used [these] for everything from shampoos to soapy water. They're cheap and come in sets."* – BHW

- Residential Heated Door Mat – *"I live in Upstate New York and we have plenty of snow and ice. After my rotator cuff surgery in the fall, I bought a heated doormat so I could get my mail and packages. It worked out pretty well."* – Dan Y. Note: Manufacturers also make longer electrical mats to keep the snow off of sidewalks.

- Passport Wallets – *"When I first started to get around I couldn't stand the thought of having a purse strap around my other shoulder, and it was impossible for me to reach around behind me or even in my pockets. I bought a nice passport wallet where I could keep a credit card or money in front of me for easy access."* – Jillian M.

- Corner Protectors – *"When my elderly mother had her surgery we were afraid of an accidental fall. She had a bed stand with sharp edges and I bought what they call silicon corner protectors just in case."* – Anonymous

19. Good Luck and Good Healing!

The Friendly Handbook of Shoulder Surgery Coping Tips and Tricks is an ongoing project. I am always looking to add tips and tricks sent to me by shoulder surgery patients. Please don't hesitate to contact me at: ShoulderingKindness@gmail.com.

I have tried to avoid brand names of products or retail store names except when they are part of a quotation. In doing my research, I found that for nearly every product mentioned, especially for kitchen and household items, there are several manufacturers. Feel free to comparison shop and choose the option you like the best. It would be valuable for future editions to get everyone's feedback on the product or brand they liked the most.

Good luck and good healing to everyone!

Made in the USA
Middletown, DE
23 July 2022

69908908R00076